How to Care for a Child with Lichen Sclerosus

A Parent's Guide to Treatment, Support, and Symptom Management

copyright © 2025 Stephanie Hinderock

All rights reserved No part of this book may be reproduced, or stored in a retrieval system, or transmitted in any form or by any means, electronic, mechanical, photocopying, recording, or otherwise, without express written permission of the publisher.

Disclaimer

By reading this disclaimer, you are accepting the terms of the disclaimer in full. If you disagree with this disclaimer, please do not read the guide.

All of the content within this guide is provided for informational and educational purposes only, and should not be accepted as independent medical or other professional advice. The author is not a doctor, physician, nurse, mental health provider, or registered nutritionist/dietician. Therefore, using and reading this guide does not establish any form of a physician-patient relationship.

Always consult with a physician or another qualified health provider with any issues or questions you might have regarding any sort of medical condition. Do not ever disregard any qualified professional medical advice or delay seeking that advice because of anything you have read in this guide. The information in this guide is not intended to be any sort of medical advice and should not be used in lieu of any medical advice by a licensed and qualified medical professional.

The information in this guide has been compiled from a variety of known sources. However, the author cannot attest to or guarantee the accuracy of each source and thus should not be held liable for any errors or omissions.

You acknowledge that the publisher of this guide will not be held liable for any loss or damage of any kind incurred as a result of this guide or the reliance on any information provided within this guide. You acknowledge and agree that you assume all risk and responsibility for any action you undertake in response to the information in this guide.

Using this guide does not guarantee any particular result (e.g., weight loss or a cure). By reading this guide, you acknowledge that there are no guarantees to any specific outcome or results you can expect.

All product names, diet plans, or names used in this guide are for identification purposes only and are the property of their respective owners. The use of these names does not imply endorsement. All other trademarks cited herein are the property of their respective owners.

Where applicable, this guide is not intended to be a substitute for the original work of this diet plan and is, at most, a supplement to the original work for this diet plan and never a direct substitute. This guide is a personal expression of the facts of that diet plan.

Where applicable, persons shown in the cover images are stock photography models and the publisher has obtained the rights to use the images through license agreements with third-party stock image companies.

Table of Contents

Introduction	**8**
What Is Lichen Sclerosus?	**10**
Causes and Symptoms	10
How It Affects Children Differently	12
The Diagnostic Journey	**14**
Finding the Right Specialist	15
What to Expect During Diagnosis	16
Dispelling Myths and Misconceptions	**18**
Understanding Common Myths About Lichen Sclerosus	18
Addressing Stigma and Misinformation	19
Helping Others Understand Your Child's Condition	20
Talking to Your Child About Lichen Sclerosus	**23**
Age-Appropriate Explanations	23
Building Trust and Openness	26
Helping Your Child Cope with Emotions	**28**
Managing Fear, Anxiety, and Frustration	28
Encouraging Resilience and Confidence	31
Building a Support Network	**35**
Working with Teachers, Coaches, and Friends	35
Finding Support Groups and Communities	38
Creating a Care Plan	**42**
Developing a Routine for Skincare and Treatment	42
Scheduling Regular Medical Checkups	45
Dietary Considerations for Kids	**49**
Foods to Support Skin Health	49
Kid-Friendly Recipes for Symptom Management	**52**
Berry Smoothie Bowl	53
Sweet Potato Fries	54
Salmon and Veggie Wraps	55

Zucchini Noodle Pasta	56
Crispy Chickpea Snack	57
Rainbow Veggie Roll-Ups	58
Oatmeal with Blueberry and Almond Toppings	59
Turkey and Avocado Lettuce Wraps	60
Mini Veggie-Loaded Egg Muffins	61
Banana and Pumpkin Seed Energy Bites	62
Preventing and Managing Flare-Ups	**64**
Recognizing Triggers	64
Quick Relief Strategies	66
Hygiene and Clothing Tips	67
Choosing the Right Products	68
Clothing and Fabric Considerations for Comfort	69
School, Social Activities, and Family Dynamics	**72**
Communicating with Teachers and Staff	72
Helping Your Child Feel Included	74
Sports and Physical Activities	74
Adapting Activities for Comfort and Safety	75
Family Dynamics	76
Looking Ahead – Adolescence and Beyond	**78**
Preparing for Puberty and Hormonal Changes	78
Transitioning to Self-Management	80
Shifting Roles as a Caregiver	82
Empowering Adolescents for Adulthood	83
Advocating for Better Awareness and Care	**85**
How to Raise Awareness in Your Community	85
Working with Medical Professionals	87
Conclusion	**91**
FAQs	**94**
References and Helpful Links	**97**

Introduction

Caring for a child with lichen sclerosus can feel overwhelming, especially for parents and caregivers new to the condition. This beginner's guide offers a clear, compassionate path to understanding and managing this chronic skin disorder in children. Lichen sclerosus is more than just a medical diagnosis—it can impact a child's physical comfort, emotional well-being, and social experiences. By learning about the condition, caregivers can provide their child with the support and treatment they need to live confidently and comfortably.

In this guide, we will talk about the following;

- What Is Lichen Sclerosus?
- The Diagnostic Journey
- Dispelling Myths and Misconceptions
- Talking to Your Child About Lichen Sclerosus
- Helping Your Child Cope with Emotions
- Building a Support Network and Creating a Care Plan
- Dietary Considerations for Kids

- Preventing and Managing Flare-Ups and Hygiene and Clothing Tips
- School and Social Activities
- Sports and Physical Activities and Family Dynamics
- Looking Ahead: Adolescence and Beyond
- Advocating for Better Awareness and Care

Keep reading to learn more about how you can support a child with lichen sclerosus and navigate the challenges that may arise along the way. By the end of this guide, you will have a better understanding of the condition and feel more equipped to provide your child with the care they deserve.

What Is Lichen Sclerosus?

Lichen sclerosus is a chronic skin condition that affects the thin, outer layer of skin, usually in the genital and anal areas. While it can occur in people of all ages and genders, it's less common in children, making a diagnosis feel confusing or unexpected for many caregivers. The condition causes patchy, white, shiny skin that can be itchy, sore, and prone to splitting. It isn't contagious, which means your child didn't "catch" it from someone else, nor can they pass it on to others.

Though the term may sound daunting, lichen sclerosus is manageable with the right treatment plan. Early intervention and consistent care play a vital role in keeping symptoms under control and preserving a child's quality of life. That's why it's essential to understand what it is and how to address your child's specific needs.

Causes and Symptoms

The cause of lichen sclerosus isn't fully understood, but studies suggest it may involve a combination of factors, including:

- ***Autoimmune responses:*** The immune system may mistakenly attack healthy skin tissue.
- ***Hormonal changes:*** Imbalances, particularly in estrogen, might trigger the condition.
- ***Genetic predisposition:*** A family history of autoimmune disorders or similar skin conditions could increase the likelihood.
- ***Skin trauma:*** Repeated friction or irritation to sensitive skin might contribute, but it doesn't directly cause the condition.

Symptoms of lichen sclerosus can vary in severity, but the most common ones include:

- Smooth, white patches of skin, often on or near the genitals or anus.
- Itching, ranging from mild to intense.
- Pain, particularly during bathroom visits, while wearing tight clothes, or during physical activities.
- Skin fragility, leading to cracking, bleeding, or pain if the skin is stretched.
- Reduced elasticity in affected areas, which can develop over time.

It's important to note that some children may not exhibit all symptoms or may only show mild signs initially. However, recognizing these early can help you seek timely medical advice.

How It Affects Children Differently

Lichen sclerosus presents unique challenges for children, as their physical and emotional development can amplify the condition's impact.

Recognizing Symptoms in Young Children

Children often lack the vocabulary to fully express discomfort. Instead of verbalizing pain or itching, they may:

- Avoid wearing certain types of clothing, like underwear or pants that feel restrictive.
- Seem hesitant or upset during bathroom routines.
- Scratch or fidget noticeably in affected areas.
- Exhibit frequent mood changes due to underlying discomfort.

These behavioral signs, combined with physical symptoms, can help you recognize when something may be wrong.

Challenges in Physical Activity

For active children, lichen sclerosus can affect their participation in sports or play. Activities that involve running, sitting for long hours, or wearing tight uniforms might become uncomfortable or even painful. Without proper intervention, this can lead to withdrawal from social and recreational opportunities.

The Emotional Toll

Children with lichen sclerosus may feel embarrassed or confused about their condition, particularly because it affects sensitive areas of the body. They might also struggle with feelings of isolation, worried that their peers or teachers won't understand what they're going through. This emotional burden can be especially pronounced in older children and teens, as they become more aware of their bodies.

Normalizing their experience and creating a supportive environment can alleviate many of these concerns. Reinforce that their condition is treatable and explain that many kids deal with medical issues—it's just a part of life.

The Diagnostic Journey

Spotting lichen sclerosus in its early stages can be challenging, especially in children. The condition often begins subtly, with mild symptoms that may be mistaken for other common skin issues, like irritation or mild eczema. However, paying close attention to persistent or unusual symptoms can help caregivers recognize when something needs further investigation.

Key early signs to watch for include:

- ***Itching:*** Your child might experience recurrent itching, particularly in the genital or anal areas, that doesn't improve with basic skincare or over-the-counter products.
- ***Skin changes:*** Look for smooth, white patches of skin that appear shiny or thinner than usual. These patches typically develop in sensitive areas but can also occur elsewhere.
- ***Discomfort during everyday activities:*** Children may avoid wearing certain clothing, complain about pain or

irritation during bathroom use, or seem unusually distressed when sitting for long periods.
- ***Behavioral clues:*** Younger children may not explain their symptoms but could exhibit behaviors like frequent scratching, avoiding physical activities, or resisting potty training.

If you notice any of these signs, it's important to keep a written log of symptoms, including when they occur and how often. This record can be extremely helpful for healthcare providers during the diagnostic process.

Finding the Right Specialist

Once you suspect lichen sclerosus, finding the right medical professional is the next step. While a pediatrician or general practitioner can be a good starting point, it's often necessary to consult with a dermatologist or a pediatric gynecologist who has experience diagnosing and treating this condition in children.

To find a specialist:

1. ***Ask for referrals:*** Your child's regular doctor can recommend specialists within your area or network. You can also ask other caregivers in support groups for recommendations.
2. ***Research credentials:*** Look for professionals who specialize in skin disorders or pediatric gynecology.

Experience with lichen sclerosus in children is especially important since it's less common in this age group.
3. ***Prepare questions:*** When booking an appointment with a specialist, make a list of questions to gauge their experience, approach, and treatment philosophy. You'll want a provider who takes the time to listen to your concerns and explain the diagnostic process clearly.

Advocating for your child is crucial. Don't hesitate to seek a second opinion if something doesn't feel right or if you're not getting the answers you need.

What to Expect During Diagnosis

The diagnostic process for lichen sclerosus can feel daunting if you're unsure what to expect. Understanding each step ahead of time can ease anxiety and help you feel more in control as a caregiver.

The Initial Appointment

At your child's first visit, the specialist will ask about their medical history and any symptoms you've observed. They may also perform a gentle physical examination, focusing on areas where symptoms are present. This can be uncomfortable for children, so explaining beforehand that the doctor is there to help can ease their worries. Some caregivers find it helpful to bring a favorite toy or item for comfort.

Diagnostic Tools

- *Visual Inspection:* Often, a trained professional can identify lichen sclerosus through a careful examination of the skin.
- *Biopsy:* If the diagnosis isn't immediately clear, the doctor may recommend a small skin biopsy. This involves taking a tiny sample of affected skin for testing. While the idea of a biopsy can sound frightening, it's generally a quick, low-risk procedure that provides valuable information.
- *Rule-Out Testing:* The specialist might also perform tests to rule out conditions with similar symptoms, like fungal infections or other skin disorders.

Follow-Up Planning

If the diagnosis confirms lichen sclerosus, the doctor will discuss the next steps with you. This may include:

- Developing a treatment plan to manage symptoms.
- Scheduling regular follow-ups to monitor progress.
- Educating you about triggers and home care to prevent flare-ups.

While the diagnostic path can feel overwhelming, catching lichen sclerosus early allows for more effective treatment and symptom management. With the right guidance and support, you'll soon feel empowered to help your child thrive despite their condition.

Dispelling Myths and Misconceptions

Despite being a relatively common condition, lichen sclerosus is often surrounded by myths and misconceptions. In this chapter, we'll address some of the most common misunderstandings and provide accurate information to help you better understand and manage your child's condition.

Understanding Common Myths About Lichen Sclerosus

Lichen sclerosus is a condition that many, including some medical professionals, may not fully understand. This lack of awareness can lead to myths and misconceptions, causing unnecessary fear or shame for caregivers and children. Clearing up these myths is key to advocating for your child and ensuring they get the care and acceptance they need.

Some common myths include:

- *"It only happens to adults."* While lichen sclerosus is more often seen in postmenopausal women, children

can still develop it. Early recognition and treatment are especially important for young patients.
- ***"It's contagious."*** This is false. Lichen sclerosus isn't caused by bacteria, a virus, or fungi and cannot be passed from person to person.
- ***"It's caused by poor hygiene or neglect."*** Another harmful myth. A child's hygiene habits don't cause lichen sclerosus. It's more likely linked to autoimmune responses, hormonal factors, or genetics.
- ***"It means something is wrong with my child's development."*** Lichen sclerosus does not interfere with a child's ability to grow or develop normally. With treatment, they can live healthy and active lives.

Understanding the science behind the condition helps caregivers combat these misconceptions and approach conversations about lichen sclerosus with confidence.

Addressing Stigma and Misinformation

Stigma often surrounds conditions affecting the skin and genitals, and lichen sclerosus is no exception. Misinformation and discomfort can lead to shame and isolation for children and caregivers. Tackling stigma begins with normalizing the conversation.

Here are some strategies to combat stigma:

1. *Educate yourself first.* Having a clear understanding of lichen sclerosus equips you to correct misinformation calmly and accurately.
2. *Be open about the condition (when appropriate).* Discussing it in a matter-of-fact way with close friends, family, or trusted caregivers like teachers can help remove unnecessary mystery or judgment.
3. *Correct misinformation gently.* If someone makes an incorrect statement or assumption, take the opportunity to educate them without hostility. For example, "Actually, lichen sclerosus isn't contagious—it's a skin condition that needs careful management."
4. *Model confidence.* Children look to their caregivers for cues on how to feel about their condition. Demonstrating acceptance and assurance can help your child feel more at peace with their diagnosis.

By breaking the cultural silence around lichen sclerosus, we create a more supportive environment for those affected by it.

Helping Others Understand Your Child's Condition

Having conversations with others about your child's lichen sclerosus might feel daunting. Whether it's talking to a teacher, coach, or family member, the goal is to foster understanding while respecting your child's privacy.

Tailor Conversations to Your Audience

How much detail you share depends on who you're speaking to and their level of involvement in your child's life. For example:

- *Teachers or school staff:* Explain how the condition affects daily activities, like sitting for long periods or bathroom routines. For example, "My child has a chronic skin condition that can cause discomfort. It's not contagious, but they may need breaks to manage symptoms."
- *Family and friends:* Close family members may have more questions, especially if they're part of your care network. Be honest but concise. "Lichen sclerosus is a condition that affects the skin. It's treatable, and with the right care, it doesn't stop [Child's Name] from doing what they love."
- *Peers or classmates (if appropriate):* Depending on your child's age and comfort level, you may craft simple explanations for peers. "It's like having really sensitive skin that needs special care."

Support Your Child in Managing Conversations

Encouraging your child to feel empowered about their condition is key. Teach them age-appropriate ways to explain it in their own words. For instance:

- A younger child might say, "It's a condition that makes my skin sensitive. I have special creams to help with it."
- An older child could use, "It's a skin condition called lichen sclerosus. It's not serious, but I have to take care of it."

Remind them it's okay to choose not to share if they feel uncomfortable. The decision of how much to disclose should always remain under their control.

Building Empathy in Others

Sometimes, people may be well-meaning but uninformed. Use these opportunities to build empathy for your child's experience. Simplify complex concepts and highlight what matters most: that your child is just like any other kid and deserves understanding and respect. Focusing on your child's strengths and resilience can help shift attention away from the condition and toward who they are as a person.

Education is the antidote to stigma and fear. By dispelling myths, addressing misinformation, and guiding others to a clearer understanding of lichen sclerosus, caregivers can create a circle of care and support that empowers their child to thrive.

Talking to Your Child About Lichen Sclerosus

As a caregiver, it can be difficult to know how to talk to your child about lichen sclerosus. You may worry about their understanding of the condition and how they will handle conversations with peers. However, open and honest communication is crucial in helping your child feel empowered and supported.

Age-Appropriate Explanations

Talking to your child about lichen sclerosus can feel intimidating, especially when the condition involves sensitive areas and symptoms that are hard to explain. The key is to tailor your conversation to their age and understanding, ensuring that explanations feel supportive rather than overwhelming.

Talking to Younger Children (Ages 3–7)

For younger kids, it's essential to keep explanations simple and focused on how things will get better. They don't need in-depth details, just reassurance that their condition is manageable.

- *Use simple language:* You could say, "You have special areas on your skin that need extra care, kind of like when you get a scrape. Mommy and the doctor have a cream to help."
- *Focus on feelings:* Ask how they're feeling when discomfort arises, and validate their emotions. For example, "I know it's itchy, and that's no fun. But I'm here to make sure it feels better quickly."
- *Reassure them:* Make it clear that they haven't done anything wrong to cause this. "This is just something that happens to some people, and it's nothing to worry about."

Talking to School-Age Children (Ages 8–12)

Children in this age group are starting to ask more questions about the world and their own bodies, so they'll likely want a bit more detail. You can gently introduce the name of the condition and explain it in more depth.

- *Introduce the condition's name:* "You have something called lichen sclerosus. It's a skin condition that can make parts of your skin sensitive or itchy, but we know how to take care of it."
- *Encourage curiosity:* If they ask why it happens, you can answer broadly without overwhelming them.

"Doctors aren't sure exactly what causes it, but we have good ways to keep it from bothering you too much."
- ***Empower them:*** Give them a role in their care. "When we put on this cream, it helps your skin stay healthy. You're doing a great job letting me know when it feels uncomfortable."

Talking to Teens

Teenagers may be more self-conscious and worried about how the condition affects their lives. It's important to approach these conversations with honesty, emphasizing their ability to manage the condition as they get older.

- ***Be open to deeper discussions:*** Teens are capable of understanding that lichen sclerosus is a chronic condition. Acknowledge, "This is something you'll need to manage, but we have treatments that work, and it doesn't have to slow you down."
- ***Address body image issues:*** They might feel embarrassed about how the condition affects their body. Assure them, "This doesn't make you any less of who you are. We're taking care of it, and it doesn't change how amazing you are."
- ***Encourage self-care:*** Start teaching them ways to manage their treatment independently, such as applying creams or recognizing symptoms of flare-ups. Giving them control promotes confidence.

Building Trust and Openness

Building trust and openness with your child early on sets the foundation for better communication about their condition as they grow. When kids feel safe sharing their thoughts and concerns, it's easier to address issues before they become overwhelming.

Create a Safe Space for Discussion

- *Be approachable:* Make sure your child knows they can come to you anytime they feel discomfort. Reassure them, "If anything feels different or bothers you, it's always okay to tell me. We'll figure it out together."
- *Listen without judgment:* When your child expresses frustration or embarrassment, validate those feelings. "I understand that this can feel hard sometimes. It's okay to feel upset."
- *Avoid overreacting:* Respond calmly to any symptoms they describe, providing reassurance rather than additional worry.

Normalize Conversations About the Body

- *Use proper terms:* Teaching anatomically correct names, especially as they relate to affected areas, reduces shame and confusion.
- *Be casual but clear:* Talk about their skin and condition like you would other health issues, such as

scrapes or colds. This normalizes it and removes the secrecy around genital or sensitive areas.
- *Answer their questions honestly:* If your child is curious, provide age-appropriate answers without evading the topic.

Support Emotional Resilience

- *Encourage self-expression:* Invite your child to talk about how they feel, whether it's frustration, worry, or curiosity.
- *Offer reassurance:* Remind them that they are not alone and that many other kids have medical conditions to manage, too.
- *Celebrate small victories:* Whether it's sticking to their routine or finding a treatment that works, acknowledge their efforts and progress.

Maintaining open communication is an ongoing effort. Keep revisiting topics as your child grows and their understanding deepens. By building a foundation of trust and openness, you help your child recognize that while their condition is part of their life, it doesn't define who they are or what they can achieve.

Helping Your Child Cope with Emotions

Children with chronic skin conditions face unique challenges that can impact their emotional well-being. From dealing with physical discomfort to managing social stigma, these factors can take a toll on a child's mental health. As a parent or caregiver, it's important to recognize and address your child's emotions in a supportive and understanding way.

Managing Fear, Anxiety, and Frustration

Living with lichen sclerosus can bring about a range of emotions for a child. They may feel fear about doctor visits, anxiety over flare-ups, or frustration with the discomfort and limitations that sometimes accompany the condition. Helping your child understand and process these emotions is a critical part of their care.

1. **Recognize and Validate Feelings**

    Children may not always have the words to express how they're feeling, so paying attention to changes in behavior or mood is important. Look for signs like withdrawal, irritability, or outbursts as clues to underlying emotional struggles.

- *Acknowledge their feelings:* Reassure your child that it's okay to feel scared, sad, or angry. You might say, "It's normal to feel upset when your skin feels uncomfortable or when we have to go to the doctor."
- *Avoid dismissing emotions:* Even if their concerns seem small, take them seriously. Saying, "You'll be fine; it's nothing to worry about," can make them feel misunderstood. Instead, offer empathy, like "I understand why this feels frustrating. It's hard to deal with sometimes."

2. **Teach Coping Skills**

Help your child build tools to handle fear and anxiety when they arise. These strategies can help them feel more in control:

- *Deep breathing exercises:* Teach your child simple breathing techniques. For example, "Breathe in like you're smelling a flower, then blow out like you're cooling soup." This can be calming during stressful moments, like doctor visits or when symptoms flare.
- *Visual imagery:* Encourage them to picture a happy, peaceful place, like their favorite park or

beach, whenever they feel scared or in pain. This mental "escape" can help distract and soothe them.
- *Use routines for reassurance:* Children thrive with consistency. Having a set routine for applying creams or taking breaks for self-care can make them feel more secure.

3. **Address Frustration in Healthy Ways**

When symptoms interfere with their activities or comfort, children may express frustration by lashing out or becoming disheartened. Support them in channeling these feelings constructively.

- *Create an outlet:* Encourage creative expression through art, journaling, or play. Drawing or writing about their feelings can help your child process them.
- *Model patience:* Show them how to handle challenges calmly by saying, "I understand this is frustrating, but we can work through it together."
- *Shift focus to solutions:* Praise them for steps they take to feel better. For example, "You did a great job telling me your skin was bothering you, and now we can make it more comfortable."

Encouraging Resilience and Confidence

Building resilience is key to helping your child thrive despite lichen sclerosus. With the proper support, they can develop the confidence to overcome challenges and maintain a positive self-image.

1. **Highlight Strengths, Not Limitations**

   Help your child see their abilities rather than focusing solely on their condition.

   - *Recognize their successes:* Celebrate achievements big and small, whether it's applying their treatment independently or excelling in a hobby.
   - *Reframe setbacks as opportunities:* If a flare-up disrupts plans, teach them to adjust. For example, "I know we had to cancel soccer today, but how about a movie night together instead?"
   - *Encourage their interests:* Support your child in pursuing activities they enjoy. This reinforces that lichen sclerosus is just one part of their life, not the whole story.

2. **Build Self-Efficacy**

   Empower your child by giving them gentle control over aspects of their care and reinforcing their ability to face challenges.

- *Teach self-care:* Depending on their age, involve them in their treatment, such as applying creams or recognizing early signs of symptoms. Independence can strengthen their confidence.
- *Use positive language:* Replace "this will always be hard" with "we're learning how to handle this better every day." Encourage a mindset of growth and resilience.

3. **Promote a Growth Mindset**

Encourage your child to see challenges as opportunities to learn and grow rather than insurmountable obstacles.

- *Tell stories of resilience:* Share age-appropriate examples of people who've overcome challenges. This could be someone in your family or even a character from a book they love.
- *Focus on effort, not perfection:* Praise their dedication to managing their condition rather than expecting flawless results. "You're doing such a good job following your treatment plan, and that's what matters most."

4. **Foster a Positive Self-Image**

   A chronic condition can sometimes make a child feel "different" from their peers. Help them understand that lichen sclerosus does not define them.

   - ***Strengthen body positivity:*** Encourage your child to appreciate everything their body does for them, even if some parts need extra care.
   - ***Use affirmations:*** Help them build confidence with phrases like "I am strong" or "I can handle tough things."
   - ***Support social experiences:*** Encourage your child to participate in social activities and friendships, which can reinforce that they are valued for who they are.

5. **Create a Safe Space for Emotional Growth**

   Ultimately, your support as a caregiver creates the foundation for your child's emotional resilience. Show them that no matter what, they have a secure base to return to.

   - Be their biggest cheerleader: Celebrate their bravery in taking on tough days.
   - Keep open communication: Check in regularly about how they're feeling and what they need from you.

- Reassure their worth: Remind them that they are loved and valued, no matter what challenges they face.

By addressing emotional challenges head-on and nurturing resilience, you can empower your child to face the ups and downs of lichen sclerosus with courage and confidence. The goal isn't to eliminate every worry but to equip them with the tools and mindset to handle whatever comes their way.

Building a Support Network

One of the most important parts of navigating life with lichen sclerosus is not doing it alone. Building a strong support network can make a huge difference for both you and your child. By working closely with teachers, coaches, friends, and finding supportive communities, you can ensure that your child feels understood, included, and empowered.

Working with Teachers, Coaches, and Friends

Many of the people in your child's life—like educators, sports coaches, and peers—can help create a positive environment where your child's needs are met. Open communication and a collaborative approach are key to helping these individuals become valuable allies.

Collaborating with Teachers

Since your child spends a significant amount of time at school, teachers play an essential role in their support system. Here's how you can work with school staff:

- ***Request a meeting:*** Schedule a discussion with your child's teacher or school nurse to explain lichen sclerosus and its impact on your child. Focus on practicalities, like symptom management during the school day.
- ***Share key information:*** Provide clear instructions on what your child might need, such as additional bathroom breaks, access to a soothing cream, or a place to rest during flare-ups.
- ***Set up accommodations:*** If needed, work with the school to create an Individualized Education Plan (IEP) or 504 Plan that addresses your child's specific requirements. This ensures their needs are documented and consistently met.
- ***Keep lines of communication open:*** Encourage regular updates. For example, check in with the teacher to see how your child is coping and if any adjustments are needed.

Partnering with Coaches and Activity Leaders

For children involved in sports or extracurricular activities, coaches and leaders can help ensure their participation is both safe and enjoyable.

- ***Explain the basics:*** You don't need to share every detail. Simply explain that your child has a condition requiring extra care and outline specific

considerations, such as avoiding friction or ensuring time for symptom management.
- ***Discuss modifications:*** Work together to adjust activities when needed. For instance, providing breaks during physical activity or helping your child find alternatives to uniforms that may irritate their skin.
- ***Promote inclusivity:*** Reinforce that your child's involvement is valuable, whether they need modifications or can fully participate. A supportive leader can model inclusivity for the entire group.

Supporting Friendships and Peers

Having understanding friends can make all the difference for your child's confidence and happiness. Encouraging positive relationships with peers helps normalize their experience and reduces the feeling of being "different."

- ***Facilitate open conversations:*** If your child is comfortable, help them explain their condition to close friends in simple terms. This can ease misunderstandings and build empathy.
- ***Playdates with purpose:*** Invite friends for activities your child enjoys and can participate in without discomfort, helping to reinforce bonds without making their condition a focal point.
- ***Encourage kindness:*** Share information about lichen sclerosus with trusted parents or caregivers within your social circle, fostering understanding and empathy.

You could say, "This just requires a little extra care, but it doesn't stop [Child's Name] from being involved in all the fun."

By working together with teachers, coaches, and friends, you create a network of people who can help your child feel safe, supported, and included, no matter where they are.

Finding Support Groups and Communities

Living with lichen sclerosus can feel isolating at times, but finding a community of people who understand your experiences can be incredibly reassuring. Both online and in-person connections can provide emotional support, practical tips, and a sense of empowerment.

1. **Locating Support Groups**

   Support groups are spaces where you can share experiences, ask for advice, and meet others who "get it." There are several ways to find these groups:

   - *Ask your healthcare provider:* Doctors or specialists may know of local or national organizations dedicated to supporting families affected by lichen sclerosus.
   - *Search online forums:* Platforms like social media or condition-specific forums often host communities where caregivers can connect to share knowledge and encouragement.

- ***Reach out to local clinics or hospitals:*** Some healthcare facilities host in-person support groups or educational sessions specifically for chronic conditions.

When joining a support group, look for one that aligns with your goals. Some may focus more on medical information, while others prioritize emotional support.

2. **Benefits of Community Support**

   Engaging with support groups and communities can provide benefits like:

   - *A safe space to share:* Discussing your experiences openly with people who understand can reduce feelings of isolation.
   - *Practical advice:* Other caregivers often have insights into managing daily challenges, from navigating school systems to finding the best products.
   - *Encouragement and positivity:* Hearing success stories and exchanging tips can remind you that you're not alone and that your child can lead a fulfilling, joyful life.

3. **Online Communities and Resources**

   The internet opens doors to a wide variety of resources. Some popular options include:

- *Condition-specific groups:* Social media platforms like Facebook often have private groups for caregivers. Search for terms like "lichen sclerosus parents" or "pediatric skin condition support."
- *Nonprofit organizations:* Many nonprofits provide online communities, webinars, or forums specifically for families managing chronic conditions. Check their websites for details.
- *Virtual meet-ups:* Some groups host scheduled online meetings, allowing you to participate from the comfort of your home.

4. **Building Your Personal Network**

Beyond formal groups, creating your own informal support network can be just as powerful. Reach out to family, friends, or other parents who can offer help or just a listening ear. Even a small circle of trusted people can make a big difference when managing care and emotions.

5. **Encouraging Your Child to Connect**

If your child expresses interest, look for groups or activities that help them connect with peers who have similar experiences. Support doesn't have to be limited to adults—kids gain incredible comfort from realizing they're not alone.

- ***Books or stories:*** Look for child-friendly books or media that emphasize acceptance and understanding of medical conditions.
- ***Workshops or camps:*** Some organizations host health-related events or programs tailored for children, giving them a chance to meet others in similar situations.

By tapping into both local and online resources, you and your child can build meaningful connections that reinforce understanding, lift spirits, and provide valuable insights.

Creating a strong support network consists of many small steps. By collaborating with the key people in your child's life and seeking out communities of caregivers and families, you establish a foundation of care for your child. These connections don't only help with practical challenges—they remind your child (and you) that you're never alone in this journey.

Creating a Care Plan

Developing a care plan for a child with lichen sclerosus is an essential step toward managing their condition effectively. A thoughtful plan helps streamline daily routines, ensures proper treatment, and provides peace of mind for caregivers and children alike. By establishing consistent skincare and scheduling regular medical checkups, you can set the foundation for long-term management and comfort.

Developing a Routine for Skincare and Treatment

Consistency is key when it comes to managing lichen sclerosus. A routine can help prevent flare-ups, reduce symptoms, and make the child feel more in control of their care.

1. **Establishing a Skincare Routine**

    Skincare is one of the cornerstones of managing lichen sclerosus. By setting up a consistent regimen, you can help protect the affected skin and alleviate discomfort.

- ***Clean Gently:*** Use a mild, fragrance-free cleanser and lukewarm water to wash the affected areas. Avoid scrubbing, as this can irritate sensitive skin. Pat the skin dry with a soft towel instead of rubbing.
- ***Apply Prescribed Treatments:*** If your doctor has recommended a topical ointment or cream (like a steroid), ensure it's applied exactly as directed. This treatment reduces inflammation, itching, and discomfort.
- ***Choose Protective Products:*** Use minimally irritating moisturizers that create a barrier to protect the skin. Look for hypoallergenic products with simple ingredients to keep sensitive areas hydrated.
- ***Dress Comfortably:*** Clothing can either help or harm the skin. Opt for loose-fitting, breathable fabrics like cotton to minimize irritation. Avoid tight waistbands or synthetic materials that might rub against sensitive areas.

2. **Building Consistency**

Fitting skincare into your child's day-to-day routine helps build consistency and reduces the chance of skipping treatments. You can weave it into times they're already familiar with, like:

- *Morning and Bedtime:* Apply creams or soothing moisturizers at the beginning and end of the day when they're naturally getting ready or winding down.
- *After Bathing:* Make post-bath your designated time for cleaning and treating the skin, ensuring the area is cared for when the skin is hydrated.
- *Using Checklists or Reminders:* Visual reminders or a chart on the bathroom wall can help kids track when they've completed a step, making them feel more engaged with their own care.

3. **Making It a Positive Experience**

Integrating care into their daily life doesn't have to feel like a chore. Create a calm and encouraging environment for skincare so your child views it as a normal part of their routine rather than something stressful.

- *Encourage Participation:* Depending on their age, allow your child to apply creams themselves with your supervision. This helps them feel independent and responsible.
- *Celebrate Small Wins:* Praise their commitment, even for little steps like remembering to wipe and apply cream after bathroom use.

- *Use Distractions When Needed:* If younger children resist, singing a song, counting, or telling a short story during application may help make the process easier.

Establishing a skincare routine not only soothes and protects their skin but also fosters a sense of empowerment as they grow into their care plan.

Scheduling Regular Medical Checkups

Routine checkups are an essential part of managing lichen sclerosus. A good partnership with your healthcare provider ensures that your child's condition is monitored, treatments are adjusted as needed, and potential complications are addressed early.

1. **Set Up Routine Appointments**

   Work with your child's doctor to define a checkup schedule. While the frequency may vary based on their symptoms and treatment, a general guideline might include:

   - *Initial Follow-Up Visits:* These might be more frequent (e.g., every 4–6 weeks) after diagnosis to assess treatment effectiveness and adjust if needed.
   - *Regular Maintenance Visits:* Once symptoms are stable, visits may be spaced out to every 3–6

months to monitor the condition and address new changes.
- *Annual Evaluations:* These comprehensive checkups allow the doctor to review long-term progress and ensure other health areas are not being impacted.

Make it a habit to jot down relevant symptoms or changes between appointments. Keeping a journal will help provide detailed updates to the physician and track progress over time.

2. Plan Ahead for Appointments

To ensure stress-free visits, preparation is key:

- *Book Early:* Schedule regular checkups in advance so you have the first pick of appointment slots that fit your child's routine.
- *Discuss Questions or Concerns:* Take a few minutes before each visit to write down any questions, new symptoms, or observations about treatments. This ensures no concerns are forgotten at the moment.
- *Pack Essentials:* Bring items to make the appointment smoother, like your child's favorite toy or snack, as well as any creams or medications currently in use for the doctor to review.

3. **Advocate for Your Child**

   During the visit, work closely with the doctor to make sure all aspects of your child's condition are addressed. Don't hesitate to:

   - *Clarify Instructions:* Ask for clear, simple explanations for any treatment changes or care recommendations.
   - *Request Resources:* If you're unsure about managing certain aspects of care, the doctor might provide brochures, videos, or online references.
   - *Explore Emerging Options:* If treatments aren't bringing the desired relief, ask about new methods or approaches that may be available.

   Your advocacy ensures your child's care stays on the right path and their needs are fully addressed.

4. **Staying on Track with Appointments**

   With all of life's responsibilities, staying on top of medical visits can be challenging. Here are tips to keep everything organized:

   - *Use a Calendar:* A physical or digital calendar (like one on your phone) can help you remember appointments and plan around them.

- ***Set Reminders:*** Many clinics now offer text reminders—take advantage of these services, or set your own phone alarms for upcoming visits.
- ***Combine Appointments:*** If your child has appointments with multiple specialists, aim to coordinate them back-to-back for convenience.

Regular medical visits, combined with your input, create a reliable framework for tracking progress and ensuring your care plan remains effective.

Creating a consistent care plan—complete with manageable daily routines and scheduled medical checkups—provides your child with the tools they need to live comfortably with lichen sclerosus. Skincare routines become part of their daily habits, while medical visits ensure their progress is regularly assessed by professionals.

Dietary Considerations for Kids

Nutrition plays a critical role in supporting overall health, including skin health, which is particularly important for children managing lichen sclerosus. While diet alone cannot cure the condition, making mindful food choices can help promote healthy skin, reduce inflammation, and support your child's overall well-being. This chapter explores foods that can benefit skin health and provides simple, kid-friendly recipes to help manage symptoms.

Foods to Support Skin Health

The right nutrients can make a difference in maintaining your child's skin barrier, calming inflammation, and ensuring they meet their overall nutritional needs. Incorporating the following types of foods into their meals can provide an added layer of support in managing their condition.

Focus on Anti-Inflammatory Foods

Since lichen sclerosus often involves inflammation, foods that naturally reduce inflammation can be helpful. Aim to include:

- *Fruits and Vegetables:* Vibrant options like berries, oranges, spinach, and sweet potatoes are packed with antioxidants that combat inflammation.
- *Healthy Fats:* Omega-3 fatty acids in foods like salmon, walnuts, chia seeds, and flaxseeds can help reduce inflammation in the body.
- *Whole Grains:* Brown rice, quinoa, and oats provide fiber, which can help reduce inflammation and support digestion.

Boost Skin Healing with Vitamins and Minerals

Certain nutrients are particularly beneficial for skin health, helping to repair and maintain its protective barrier:

- *Vitamin A:* Found in carrots, sweet potatoes, and leafy greens, it promotes healthy skin cell growth.
- *Vitamin C:* This powerful antioxidant, present in citrus fruits, strawberries, and bell peppers, aids in collagen production and wound healing.
- *Vitamin E:* Found in almonds, sunflower seeds, and avocados, it helps protect skin cells and retain moisture.
- *Zinc:* Found in beans, nuts, and fortified cereals, zinc can assist with skin repair and reduce inflammation.

Stay Hydrated

Hydration is vital for keeping skin supple and reducing dryness, so encourage your child to drink water throughout the day. Foods with high water content, like cucumbers, watermelon, and oranges, can also contribute to hydration.

Avoid Trigger Foods

While every child is different, some foods may worsen inflammation or sensitivities for certain kids. These might include:

- ***Refined Sugars:*** Found in candy, baked goods, and sugary drinks, they can contribute to inflammation.
- ***Processed Foods:*** Snack chips, fast food, and packaged meals may include additives that irritate sensitive systems.
- ***Dairy or Gluten (if reactive):*** While not every child with lichen sclerosus needs to avoid these, some find relief by eliminating potential triggers. Keep a food diary if you suspect certain foods may be causing flare-ups.

By focusing on nutrient-dense, whole foods and minimizing irritants, you create a diet that supports your child's body as it manages the challenges of lichen sclerosus.

Kid-Friendly Recipes for Symptom Management

Healthy meals don't have to be complicated! Here are some simple, delicious recipes designed to prioritize nutrients while keeping kids happy.

Berry Smoothie Bowl

Packed with antioxidants and vitamins, this colorful smoothie bowl is both a treat and a nutritional powerhouse.

Ingredients:

- 1 frozen banana
- 1/2 cup frozen mixed berries (blueberries, raspberries, or strawberries)
- 1/2 cup unsweetened almond milk (or any non-dairy milk, if preferred)
- 1 tablespoon ground flaxseeds or chia seeds
- Toppings (optional): sliced fresh fruits, granola, or coconut flakes

Instructions:

1. Blend banana, berries, almond milk, and flaxseeds until smooth.
2. Pour into a bowl and add your child's favorite toppings.

Why it's good: Berries are rich in antioxidants, while the flaxseeds provide omega-3 fatty acids for inflammation support.

Sweet Potato Fries

These baked fries are a delicious, nutrient-rich alternative to traditional fries.

Ingredients:

- 2 medium sweet potatoes, sliced into wedges
- 1 tablespoon olive oil
- 1 teaspoon paprika
- 1/2 teaspoon garlic powder
- Salt to taste

Instructions:

1. Preheat the oven to 425°F (220°C).
2. Toss sweet potato wedges in olive oil, paprika, garlic powder, and salt.
3. Spread in a single layer on a baking sheet lined with parchment paper.
4. Bake for 20-25 minutes, flipping halfway through, until golden and crispy.

Why it's good: Sweet potatoes are loaded with vitamin A, which supports skin health and immune function.

Salmon and Veggie Wraps

This simple wrap is packed with omega-3s and fresh veggies for a skin-nourishing meal.

Ingredients:

- 1 whole-grain tortilla or gluten-free wrap
- 1 small cooked salmon fillet (or canned salmon, drained)
- 1/4 avocado, sliced
- 1/4 cup shredded carrots
- A handful of spinach or arugula leaves
- 1 tablespoon hummus (optional)

Instructions:

1. Lay the tortilla flat and spread hummus (if using).
2. Add salmon, avocado slices, carrots, and spinach to the center.
3. Roll it up tightly and cut it into smaller pieces for easy handling.

Why it's good: Salmon provides essential omega-3 fatty acids, while spinach and carrots add vitamins and minerals for skin repair.

Zucchini Noodle Pasta

A fun way for kids to enjoy veggies, this pasta swap is both tasty and light on inflammation triggers.

Ingredients:

- 2 medium zucchinis (use a spiralizer or buy pre-cut zucchini noodles)
- 1 cup marinara sauce (look for a low-sugar, natural brand)
- 1 tablespoon olive oil
- 1/4 cup grated Parmesan or nutritional yeast (optional)

Instructions:

1. Heat olive oil in a pan over medium heat. Sauté zucchini noodles for 2-3 minutes until just tender.
2. Add marinara sauce and warm through.
3. Serve with grated Parmesan or nutritional yeast, if desired.

Why it's good: Zucchini is hydrating and packed with vitamins, while the olive oil supports anti-inflammatory benefits.

Crispy Chickpea Snack

This high-protein snack is perfect for on-the-go munching and adds a satisfying crunch to their day.

Ingredients:

- 1 can chickpeas, drained and rinsed
- 1 tablespoon olive oil
- 1 teaspoon cumin
- 1/4 teaspoon salt

Instructions:

1. Preheat the oven to 400°F (200°C).
2. Toss chickpeas in olive oil, cumin, and salt. Spread them on a baking sheet.
3. Bake for 20-25 minutes, shaking the pan halfway through, until golden and crunchy.

Why it's good: Chickpeas are rich in zinc, which supports skin repair and immune health.

Rainbow Veggie Roll-Ups

These colorful roll-ups are a fun way to sneak in veggies while providing a variety of vitamins and antioxidants.

Ingredients:

- 1 whole-grain tortilla or gluten-free wrap
- 2 tablespoons cream cheese or hummus
- 1 small carrot, grated
- 1/2 red bell pepper, thinly sliced
- A handful of spinach or kale leaves
- 1/4 cucumber, sliced into thin strips

Instructions:

1. Spread cream cheese or hummus over the tortilla.
2. Layer the veggies evenly across the wrap.
3. Roll up tightly and slice into pinwheels.

Why it's good: This recipe is packed with a variety of vitamins like A, C, and K, which help nourish and repair the skin.

Oatmeal with Blueberry and Almond Toppings

A warm, comforting breakfast that supports skin health with a perfect balance of whole grains, antioxidants, and healthy fats.

Ingredients:

- 1 cup rolled oats
- 2 cups unsweetened almond milk or water
- 1/2 cup fresh or frozen blueberries
- 1 tablespoon almond butter
- 1 teaspoon honey or maple syrup (optional)

Instructions:

1. Cook oats in almond milk or water according to package instructions.
2. Top with blueberries, a dollop of almond butter, and a drizzle of honey if desired.

Why it's good: Whole oats contain zinc and antioxidants, while blueberries provide powerful anti-inflammatory benefits, and almonds add vitamin E.

Turkey and Avocado Lettuce Wraps

These wraps are high in protein and healthy fats to support skin repair and overall health.

Ingredients:

- 4 large romaine or butter lettuce leaves
- 1 cup cooked ground turkey or turkey slices
- 1/2 avocado, sliced
- 1 small tomato, diced
- 1 tablespoon olive oil
- A pinch of salt and pepper

Instructions:

1. Lay lettuce leaves flat and fill each with turkey, avocado, and tomato.
2. Drizzle with olive oil and sprinkle with salt and pepper.
3. Fold or roll up and serve.

Why it's good: Turkey provides protein, which helps with skin repair, while avocado and olive oil include healthy fats that boost hydration and reduce inflammation.

Mini Veggie-Loaded Egg Muffins

Perfect for breakfast or snacks, these mini egg muffins are full of nutrients and easy to prep ahead.

Ingredients:

- 4 large eggs
- 1/2 cup chopped spinach
- 1/4 cup diced bell peppers
- 1/4 cup shredded cheese (optional)
- A pinch of salt and pepper

Instructions:

1. Preheat the oven to 375°F (190°C) and grease a muffin tin.
2. Whisk the eggs in a bowl, then stir in the spinach, bell peppers, cheese, along with a pinch of salt and pepper.
3. Distribute the egg mixture evenly into the muffin cups, filling each to about three-quarters of its capacity.
4. Bake for 15–20 minutes or until fully set.

Why it's good: Eggs are packed with nutrients like protein, vitamin D, and selenium, which support healthy skin, while the veggies provide additional antioxidants.

Banana and Pumpkin Seed Energy Bites

These no-bake bites are a great grab-and-go snack that combines skin-supporting nutrients with kid-friendly flavors.

Ingredients:

- 1 ripe banana, mashed
- 1/2 cup rolled oats
- 2 tablespoons pumpkin seeds
- 1 tablespoon honey
- 1 tablespoon chia seeds
- 1/4 teaspoon cinnamon

Instructions:

1. Mash the banana in a mixing bowl.
2. Add oats, pumpkin seeds, honey, chia seeds, and cinnamon, mixing until fully combined.
3. Roll mixture into small balls (about a tablespoon each) and refrigerate for at least 30 minutes.

Why it's good: Pumpkin seeds are rich in zinc for skin repair, while chia seeds offer omega-3s for reducing inflammation. The banana adds natural sweetness and potassium.

Encouraging healthy eating habits takes time, but these small changes can make a big difference in your child's overall well-being. Offer colorful, nutrient-dense foods throughout the day and involve your child in meal planning or preparation whenever possible. This not only empowers them but can also spark enthusiasm about nutritious choices.

Remember, while these dietary tips and recipes support skin health, they work best as part of a broader care plan. Combine them with consistent skincare routines, regular medical checkups, and emotional support to help your child manage lichen sclerosus with confidence and ease.

Preventing and Managing Flare-Ups

Managing lichen sclerosus involves more than just treatment; it's about understanding what can cause flare-ups and taking proactive steps to minimize discomfort. Flare-ups, or periods when symptoms worsen, can be frustrating for children and caregivers alike. This chapter provides practical advice on recognizing and avoiding triggers, managing discomfort quickly, and making thoughtful choices around hygiene, clothing, and products to support your child's comfort and well-being.

Recognizing Triggers

Understanding what causes flare-ups is the first step toward prevention. Common triggers vary from child to child, but being observant and keeping track of patterns can help pinpoint what might be exacerbating symptoms.

Common Triggers to Watch For:

- ***Irritating Products:*** Fragrances, dyes, and harsh chemicals in soaps, shampoos, and laundry detergents can irritate sensitive skin.
- ***Tight Clothing:*** Clothing that rubs or puts pressure on sensitive areas can lead to outbreaks and discomfort.
- ***Specific Foods (if sensitive):*** While rare, some children may notice a link between their diet and symptoms, such as with dairy, gluten, or processed sugar.
- ***Stress:*** Emotional stress can sometimes trigger physical symptoms. Anxiety about school, social situations, or even health concerns might play a part in flare-ups.
- ***Environmental Factors:*** Hot and humid weather, or very dry, cold conditions, can affect the skin's balance and cause flares.

Keeping a Symptom Journal

A journal can help caregivers identify patterns and potential triggers. Include details like:

- Foods consumed
- Clothing choices
- Hygiene products used
- Emotional changes (e.g., stress levels)
- Recent environmental factors (e.g., weather or activities)

By noting flare-ups alongside daily habits, you may find actionable insights into how to better manage your child's symptoms.

Quick Relief Strategies

Even with precautionary measures, flare-ups can still happen. Having strategies in place can make it easier to manage symptoms quickly and get your child back to feeling more comfortable.

Steps to Take During a Flare-Up:

1. *Cool Compress:* A clean, damp cloth or ice pack wrapped in a soft towel can help reduce itching or burning. Avoid applying ice directly to the skin.
2. *Apply Medications:* If prescribed a steroid cream or soothing ointment, apply it as directed by your healthcare provider.
3. *Use a Gentle Barrier Cream:* Products containing zinc oxide or petroleum jelly can protect irritated skin from further friction.
4. *Encourage Rest:* Physical activity, like running or sports, can worsen symptoms during a flare-up. Suggest quiet activities that allow the skin to recover.
5. *Hydration and Diet:* Encourage your child to drink water and offer nutrient-rich foods that help fight inflammation, such as fruits and vegetables.

Discuss quick-relief approaches with your child's doctor to ensure you're confident in applying these strategies when needed.

Hygiene and Clothing Tips

Taking extra care with daily hygiene and clothing choices is an essential part of managing lichen sclerosus. These small adjustments can go a long way in preventing flare-ups and promoting comfort.

Hygiene Tips:

- ***Gentle Cleansing:*** Use lukewarm water and fragrance-free, hypoallergenic cleansers for bathing. Avoid scrubbing sensitive areas; instead, gently pat the skin clean.
- ***Daily Care:*** Incorporate your child's prescribed creams into their routine and apply after bathing to lock in hydration.
- ***Avoid Irritants:*** Skip bubble baths, harsh soaps, and scented wipes. Use moist, unscented wipes if needed for cleansing.

Bathing as a Comfort Tool:

Consider short sits in a lukewarm bath with a tablespoon of baking soda or oatmeal powder to soothe itching and inflammation.

Daily Clothing Suggestions:

Comfort starts with choosing the right fabrics and fit. Use the following tips to keep your child comfortable:

- Loose-fitting clothing reduces friction on sensitive skin.
- Opt for breathable, natural fabrics like 100% cotton.
- Avoid tight elastic bands on underwear or pants that might create pressure on affected areas.

Choosing the Right Products

The products you use in your child's daily routines play a major role in skin health. Products that are too harsh or contain unnecessary ingredients can worsen symptoms.

What to Look For:

- *Fragrance-Free and Dye-Free:* Whether it's soap, shampoo, or laundry detergent, select products labeled for sensitive skin with no added fragrances or dyes.
- *Moisturizing Properties:* Cleansers should include soothing ingredients like glycerin or aloe to maintain the skin's natural barrier.
- *Hypoallergenic and Gentle Ingredients:* Products that are dermatologist-tested for sensitive skin can reduce the risk of irritant reactions.

Laundry Detergent Tips:
- Use a mild, hypoallergenic detergent without fragrances.
- Double rinse your child's clothes to remove any soap residue.

Simple swaps in everyday care routines can drastically reduce the likelihood of triggering symptoms with irritating products.

Clothing and Fabric Considerations for Comfort

Being thoughtful about what your child wears is just as important as skin treatments. The right clothing can prevent unnecessary irritation and keep flare-ups at bay.

Prioritize Comfortable Fabrics:

Natural and breathable materials are ideal for children with lichen sclerosus:

- *Cotton:* Soft, airy, and gentle on the skin.
- *Bamboo:* Lightweight and naturally moisture-wicking.
- *Modal:* A smooth, breathable material ideal for sensitive skin.

On the flip side, you'll want to avoid synthetic fabrics like polyester or nylon, which can trap heat and moisture, potentially leading to irritation.

Pay Attention to Fit:

Your child's clothes should:

- Allow plenty of movement without rubbing affected areas.
- Be tag-free or have soft seams to avoid irritating delicate skin.
- Include underwear that fits snugly but doesn't press tightly against the groin area.

Seasonal Adjustments:

- *Summer:* Loose clothing, sun hats, and breathable fabrics can prevent sweat-related discomfort.
- *Winter:* Avoid harsh wool or heavy layers directly on the skin; opt for light cotton as a base layer to avoid scratching or redness.

By building a wardrobe that prioritizes comfort and functionality, you can ensure fewer external factors lead to unnecessary stress on your child's skin.

Preventing and managing flare-ups may feel daunting at first, but with a combination of vigilance and thoughtful care, it's possible to create a stable routine that reduces their frequency and severity. Recognizing triggers, providing quick relief, and fine-tuning hygiene and clothing habits offer your child daily comfort and protection.

You're not just easing symptoms; you're creating an environment that helps your child feel in control and cared for. By staying proactive and adaptable, you can empower both yourself and your child to manage lichen sclerosus with confidence and comfort.

School, Social Activities, and Family Dynamics

Helping a child with lichen sclerosus thrive goes beyond medical care—it involves navigating school life, social activities, and family relationships with thoughtfulness and care. In this chapter, we'll explore how caregivers can advocate for their child at school, help them feel included in social settings, adapt activities to suit their needs, and maintain a healthy family dynamic.

We'll also focus on the importance of self-care for parents, recognizing that your well-being is essential in supporting your child.

Communicating with Teachers and Staff

Effective communication with your child's educators and school staff can create an environment where their needs are understood and supported.

Tips for Talking to Teachers and Staff:

- **Schedule a Meeting Early On**

    Meet with your child's teacher, school nurse, and other relevant staff to explain their diagnosis and how it may impact them in school.

- **Share Key Information**

    Provide a list of triggers, symptoms to watch for, and strategies that help if your child experiences discomfort. For instance, they may need extra restroom breaks or a private space to reapply medication.

- **Advocate for Accommodations**

    Explore options like a 504 Plan if your child needs specific accommodations, such as wearing loose-fitting clothing or sitting on a cushion.

- **Build a Support Plan**

    Collaborate with staff to create a plan for managing flare-ups at school. Ensure they know whom to contact if your child is in pain or discomfort.

Educating those in your child's school community fosters understanding and ensures your child feels safe and cared for.

Helping Your Child Feel Included

Social inclusion is an important part of childhood, but chronic conditions like lichen sclerosus can sometimes make children feel different.

Normalize Their Experience

Explain to your child, in age-appropriate language, that many kids deal with health challenges and that it's okay to talk about their condition if they want to.

Role-Playing Social Scenarios

Practice how they might respond to questions or situations where they feel self-conscious. For example, they can say, "I have sensitive skin, so I have to be careful."

Arrange Playdates

Organize small gatherings with friends who understand and support your child. This can help them build confidence in social settings.

When kids feel included and supported, they're more likely to enjoy a positive and fulfilling social life.

Sports and Physical Activities

Remaining active is important for children's physical and emotional well-being, but some sports or activities might need adjustments to ensure your child's comfort.

Choosing Suitable Sports

Opt for activities with minimal friction or tight uniforms, such as swimming, where loose-fitting swimsuits can be worn. Other low-impact options like yoga or dance may also work well.

Requesting Modifications

Speak with coaches to allow modifications like wearing softer gear or taking breaks when needed. For instance, your child might wear breathable shorts under their uniform for added comfort.

Active participation in sports promotes physical strength, reduces stress, and helps your child connect with peers.

Adapting Activities for Comfort and Safety

From school events to family outings, some activities may require minor tweaks to accommodate your child's needs.

1. *Seating Options:* For long events, bring a soft cushion or portable seat to minimize discomfort.
2. *Extra Outfits:* Carry spare clothing in case your child gets sweaty or uncomfortable.
3. *Sun Protection:* Use hats, loose clothing, and sunscreen to shield sensitive skin during outdoor events.

4. *Travel Preparedness:* Pack essential items like medication, soothing creams, and wipes when attending events away from home.

Thoughtful planning makes it easier for your child to participate fully while staying comfortable.

Family Dynamics

Living with lichen sclerosus can affect the entire household, and maintaining stability within family dynamics is key to long-term success.

Supporting Siblings and Managing Family Stress

Siblings might feel overlooked or struggle to understand why their sibling needs special attention. Open communication and shared experiences can help ease these feelings.

- *Have One-on-One Moments:* Set aside time for siblings to ensure they feel valued and heard.
- *Explain the Condition:* Use age-appropriate language to help siblings understand what lichen sclerosus is and how they can support their sibling.
- *Encourage Cooperation:* Frame family routines as a team effort, involving everyone in creating a supportive environment.

Empathy and understanding among family members can help reduce tension and strengthen relationships.

Self-Care for Parents

Caring for a child with a chronic condition is demanding. Without taking steps to care for yourself, caregiver fatigue can lead to burnout.

Tips for Prioritizing Your Well-Being:

1. *Set Boundaries:* Take time for yourself without guilt. Whether it's reading a book, exercising, or pursuing a hobby, make self-care a non-negotiable.
2. *Reach Out for Help:* Lean on support groups, friends, or family members for assistance and emotional support.
3. *Practice Stress Management:* Techniques like mindfulness, yoga, or journaling can help manage stress.
4. *Celebrate Small Wins:* Acknowledge and celebrate the progress your child makes, as well as your role in fostering their growth.

When parents care for themselves, they're better equipped to support their child and maintain a healthy family dynamic.

School, social activities, and family life all play a critical role in helping your child build confidence and manage their condition. By maintaining open communication with educators, adapting activities thoughtfully, and addressing family needs with care, you create a strong, united framework for success.

Looking Ahead – Adolescence and Beyond

As children with lichen sclerosus grow older, they face new experiences that bring both opportunities and challenges. Adolescence is a period of significant physical, emotional, and social changes. For those managing lichen sclerosus, these changes can feel even more pronounced.

This chapter focuses on preparing for puberty and hormonal changes, while also guiding caregivers and teens on transitioning toward greater independence in self-managing their condition. By fostering open communication and building essential skills, you can help your child approach this next phase with confidence.

Preparing for Puberty and Hormonal Changes

The hormonal fluctuations of puberty can influence skin conditions, including lichen sclerosus. It's important for both caregivers and adolescents to understand how these changes may affect symptoms, so they feel prepared and empowered to manage them.

1. **What to Expect During Puberty:**
   - *Hormonal Shifts:* Changes in hormone levels can lead to flare-ups for some teens, while others may notice minimal to no difference in their symptoms.
   - *Growth in Self-Awareness:* Adolescents may become more conscious of their body, including symptoms like itching or scarring. This awareness can sometimes lead to feelings of self-consciousness or emotional stress.
   - *Changes in Routine Needs:* Puberty may necessitate adjustments to skincare routines, such as increased use of moisturizers or specific hygiene practices.
2. **How Caregivers Can Support Their Child:**
   - *Start the Conversation Early:* Begin discussing puberty and its potential effects on lichen sclerosus before the changes begin. Use age-appropriate language to reduce anxiety and confusion.
   - *Educate About Reproductive Health:* Teach them about the importance of protecting sensitive areas and being mindful of changes. If your child is female, this includes

understanding how their condition might interact with menstrual care and vaginal health.
- ***Encourage Body Positivity:*** Normalize and celebrate their individuality. Remind them that everyone's body experiences changes, and teach them to view their own with understanding and care.
- ***Connect With Specialists:*** During puberty, regular follow-ups with a dermatologist or gynecologist (if applicable) can provide professional guidance and reassure your teen about their health.

Preparing your child for these transitions builds their confidence and helps them view puberty as a natural step forward rather than a daunting hurdle.

Transitioning to Self-Management

Adolescence is also a time to begin gradually transferring responsibility for managing lichen sclerosus from caregiver to child. This transition equips them with the tools they'll need to live independently while maintaining control over their condition.

1. **Steps for Gradual Self-Management:**
    - ***Educate on Their Condition:*** Make sure your teen understands their diagnosis, including what triggers flare-ups, why their skincare and

treatment routines are necessary, and how medications work.

- ***Teach Practical Skills:*** Walk through daily routines like applying medications, tracking symptoms, and managing flare-ups. Practicing these tasks together builds their confidence.
- ***Encourage Responsibility Over Time:*** Gradually step back by assigning small tasks they can handle alone, such as packing their medication for outings or scheduling their own reminders for treatments.

2. **Building a Symptom Tracking Habit:**

Encouraging adolescents to keep a symptom journal is a useful step toward independence. Show them how to log triggers, reactions to products, and the success of treatments. Apps designed for health tracking can also modernize this process in a way teens enjoy.

3. **Supporting Emotional Readiness:**

Self-management isn't just about the practical side—it's also about emotional resilience. Remind them that it's okay to face setbacks and to ask for help when they need it. Building this mindset encourages self-compassion and reduces frustration as they take on new responsibilities.

4. **Helping Prepare for Doctor Visits:**

   Teach your child how to advocate for themselves in medical settings by practicing how to describe symptoms or ask questions. Over time, they'll feel more comfortable voicing their needs directly to healthcare providers.

Shifting Roles as a Caregiver

While adolescence marks the start of your child's self-management, your role doesn't disappear—it simply evolves.

1. **Maintaining a Supportive Presence:**
   - Continue providing emotional support and encouragement as they take on more responsibility.
   - Stay involved in medical appointments, particularly if they ask for guidance, but give them room to take the lead.
   - Be a constant source of reassurance; remind them they don't have to have all the answers right away.
2. **Offering Guidance When Needed:**

   Even as your teen becomes more independent, there will be times when they may need extra help, such as during flare-ups or stressful life events. Lean into these moments as opportunities to reinforce their skills and remind them of your ongoing support.

Empowering Adolescents for Adulthood

Adolescence is not only about managing the present—it's also about equipping teens with the tools they'll need for their adult lives. By the time they grow into adulthood, they should feel capable of managing their condition independently.

1. **Key Skills for the Future:**
    - *Understanding Treatments:* Make sure they know how to refill prescriptions, read medication labels, and recognize when it's time to consult a doctor.
    - *Building a Support Network:* Teach them how to share information about their condition with trusted individuals, whether friends or future partners, so their social and emotional needs are met.
    - *Learning to Handle Stress:* Introducing stress management strategies, like mindfulness or exercise, can help them balance emotional challenges, which often arise during adolescence.

The goal is to empower your teen to manage their condition with confidence. By providing them with the necessary skills and support, you can help them build a strong foundation for their future as independent adults.

Advocating for Better Awareness and Care

When it comes to supporting a child with lichen sclerosus, advocacy plays a powerful role. Raising awareness within your community and collaborating with medical professionals can pave the way for better understanding, improved care, and access to resources. This chapter will focus on how caregivers can become proactive champions for their child's needs while contributing to the larger goal of increasing awareness about lichen sclerosus.

How to Raise Awareness in Your Community

Raising awareness about lichen sclerosus in your community helps to reduce stigma, foster understanding, and build a support network. By educating others, you create an environment where your child can feel seen and supported.

1. **Starting the Conversation**

   Sometimes, the simplest conversations make the biggest impact. Start small by talking to people in your immediate circle—friends, family members, or other parents. Explain the condition in clear, relatable terms and focus on what it means for your child.

For example, you might say, "Lichen sclerosus is a rare skin condition that can cause irritation and itching. My child has it, and we manage it with treatments, but it's something we have to be mindful of every day."

2. **Using Local Platforms**

Leverage local groups and resources to spread awareness further. Consider these ideas:

- *Social Media:* If you feel comfortable, share educational posts or articles on your social media. You don't need to focus on personal details—general information can go a long way.
- *Community Events:* Organize or participate in local health fairs or parent meet-ups to provide information about lichen sclerosus. Offering pamphlets or a quick talk can help others learn.
- *School Programs:* Work with your child's school to provide educational sessions for teachers, nurses, or parents. Focus on the importance of understanding sensitive health conditions.

3. **Sharing Stories**

Personal stories resonate with people and can make medical conditions more relatable. If you're comfortable, share your family's experiences, focusing on what you've learned and how others can help. You never know—someone in your community may also be facing a similar challenge and feel relief knowing they're not alone.

4. Collaborating With Support Groups

Many families dealing with lichen sclerosus feel isolated. Joining or starting a local support group for caregivers or individuals dealing with the condition fosters connection and learning. Online forums and social media groups are also excellent spaces to share ideas and resources.

Even small actions like these contribute to normalizing discussions around lichen sclerosus and ensuring caregivers don't feel they're navigating this path alone.

Working with Medical Professionals

Healthcare providers are key partners in managing lichen sclerosus. Fostering a positive, collaborative relationship with them ensures better outcomes for your child while helping to improve care on a larger scale.

1. Building a Partnership with Healthcare Providers

Advocating for your child involves creating a strong partnership with doctors, nurses, and specialists. Here's how you can foster effective communication:

- ***Be Open and Honest:*** Share all relevant details about your child's symptoms, triggers, and emotional well-being. This helps the doctor create a more personalized care plan.
- ***Ask Questions:*** If something is unclear, ask. For example, "How will this medication help my child?" or "Are there other treatments we should consider?" Getting clarity strengthens your role as an advocate.
- ***Share Observations:*** Bring notes or symptom logs to appointments. These can provide valuable insights and ensure the doctor has a complete picture of what your child is experiencing.

2. **Advocating for a Second Opinion**

   If you feel your child's needs are not being met, don't hesitate to seek a second opinion. It's your right to ensure your child gets the best possible care. Explain your concerns politely and clearly, such as, "I'd like another perspective on managing flare-ups, as we haven't seen much improvement."

3. **Promoting Awareness Within Medical Communities**

   While many medical professionals are familiar with lichen sclerosus, some may not fully understand its nuances. If you encounter this, you can help raise awareness by:

- ***Sharing Research:*** Have copies of reputable articles or studies on lichen sclerosus available, especially if your doctor seems unfamiliar with new treatment options.
- ***Suggesting Specialist Referrals:*** If your general practitioner isn't well-versed in lichen sclerosus care, request referrals to specialists such as dermatologists or pediatric gynecologists.

Your advocacy doesn't just support your child—it contributes to better understanding and treatment for others managing the same condition.

4. **Raising Awareness with Healthcare Institutions**

If you're passionate about broader advocacy, consider reaching out to hospitals or medical practices. For example:

- Offer to share your knowledge with healthcare providers through panels or discussions.
- Suggest making educational materials about lichen sclerosus available in waiting rooms or on clinic websites.

When more healthcare professionals are informed, individuals living with lichen sclerosus benefit from earlier diagnoses and improved care options.

Advocacy isn't about taking on the world—it's about taking one small step at a time. Whether you're spreading awareness in your community or building partnerships with medical professionals, each action has the potential to make a positive impact.

By educating others, collaborating with experts, and amplifying the voices of families navigating lichen sclerosus, you become a catalyst for better care and understanding. These efforts create a ripple effect, shaping a world where individuals living with lichen sclerosus feel seen, validated, and supported every step of the way.

Conclusion

Thank you for taking the time to read this guide on lichen sclerosus. By reaching the end, you've already taken a significant step toward supporting your child's health and well-being. Caring for a child with a chronic condition can feel overwhelming at first, but with the right tools, strategies, and mindset, you're more than capable of navigating this with grace and confidence.

Lichen sclerosus may be part of your child's life, but it doesn't define who they are—or who you are as a caregiver. This guide has equipped you with essential knowledge, from understanding the condition itself to managing it through daily routines, dietary considerations, and emotional support. More importantly, it's provided you with insights on how to foster resilience, not just in your child, but in yourself and your family as well.

Managing this condition isn't just about treatment plans and doctor visits—it's about building an environment of understanding and support. It's about recognizing that every small step, whether it's a flare-up avoided, a healthy meal made, or a meaningful conversation had, contributes to your child's ability to thrive. Your efforts are vital and impactful, even when progress feels slow or the challenges seem daunting.

Remember, you're not alone in this. There's an entire community of caregivers, families, and healthcare professionals working toward the same goal. By connecting with these networks, sharing your experiences, and seeking out resources, you're helping to create a better world not only for your child but also for others living with lichen sclerosus. Lean into these relationships—they are just as important as any treatment plan.

It's also worth emphasizing how powerful knowledge is. By understanding the triggers, treatment options, and daily strategies, you're becoming an expert advocate for your child. Your role as their advocate builds a bridge between their needs and the support they receive from teachers, peers, and medical professionals. This advocacy doesn't just help your child—it contributes to greater awareness and improved care across the board.

Caregiving, while rewarding, can take a toll. Don't forget to care for yourself, too. Prioritize your own well-being and remind yourself that it's okay to ask for help or take a break. By supporting yourself, you'll be better equipped to support your child and the rest of your family.

Above all, celebrate the victories big and small. Every step forward is a testament to your dedication and your child's strength. Whether it's managing a successful school day, teaching your child to apply their medication independently, or simply sharing a laugh together, these moments matter.

This guide is just the beginning. Your willingness to learn, adapt, and grow alongside your child ensures that they can face the road ahead with confidence. Continue to seek out knowledge, share your story, and advocate for better understanding and care. Together, we can create a future where lichen sclerosus is met with the understanding and compassion it deserves.

FAQs

What is lichen sclerosus, and how does it affect children?

Lichen sclerosus is a chronic skin condition causing smooth, white patches, often in the genital or anal areas. It can lead to itching, soreness, and sensitivity, making daily activities uncomfortable for children. While not contagious, it needs ongoing care to manage symptoms and prevent complications. Early diagnosis and consistent treatment can help children thrive.

What should I do if I suspect my child has lichen sclerosus?

If your child has symptoms like persistent itching, white skin patches, or discomfort during activities or using the bathroom, see a doctor. A specialist, like a dermatologist or pediatric gynecologist, can usually diagnose it with a physical exam or, in rare cases, a small skin biopsy. Keeping a symptom journal can also help the doctor with an accurate diagnosis and treatment plan.

How can I help my child manage flare-ups effectively?

During a flare-up, focus on soothing symptoms. Apply prescribed creams or ointments, use a cool compress or a soothing bath with baking soda or oatmeal, and encourage rest. Avoiding triggers like tight clothing, fragrances, or certain foods can help reduce symptoms. Keep communication open with your child to respond quickly to their discomfort.

What practical steps can I take to avoid triggering symptoms?

Choose loose, breathable cotton clothing to minimize triggers. Use fragrance-free, dye-free skincare and laundry products. Skip bubble baths and harsh soaps, and ensure your child's routine includes gentle washing and moisturizing. A consistent care routine helps control symptoms and reduce discomfort.

How do I talk to my child about lichen sclerosus without overwhelming them?

Adjust the conversation to your child's age. For younger kids, say "your skin needs special care, like a scratch," and reassure them it's not their fault. For older kids or teens, use simple terms to explain the condition and involve them in their care to help them feel in control. Keep the tone positive and remind them their condition doesn't define them.

How can I ensure my child feels included despite their condition?

Encouragement and preparation are key. Help your child join school activities or sports by sharing their needs with teachers and coaches, like bathroom breaks or extra time for self-care. Role-play social situations to build their confidence in explaining their condition if they want to. Surround them with supportive friends and peers.

What should I discuss with my child's healthcare provider during appointments?

During medical visits, share any changes in symptoms, triggers, or treatment responses. Ask about new therapies, long-term plans, and what to expect as your child grows. If you're unsure, ask for clarification—health care providers are there to help. Keeping a list of concerns ensures nothing gets missed.

References and Helpful Links

Ventolini, G., Patel, R., & Vasquez, R. (2015). Lichen sclerosus: a potpourri of misdiagnosed cases based on atypical clinical presentations. International Journal of Women S Health, 511. https://doi.org/10.2147/ijwh.s82879

Lichen sclerosus in children: care instructions. (n.d.). https://myhealth.alberta.ca/Health/aftercareinformation/pages/conditions.aspx?hwid=acd6463

Lichen sclerosus - Symptoms and causes. (n.d.). Mayo Clinic. https://www.mayoclinic.org/diseases-conditions/lichen-sclerosus/symptoms-causes/syc-20374448

Jaclyn. (2022, February 5). How to help children affected by pediatric Lichen sclerosus. Lichen Sclerosus Support Network. https://www.lssupport.net/how-to-help-children-affected-by-pediatric-lichen-sclerosus/

Kids Health Info : Lichen sclerosus. (n.d.). https://www.rch.org.au/kidsinfo/fact_sheets/Lichen_sclerosus/

MacPherson, R., & Nikolay_Donetsk/iStock/GettyImages. (2021, August 6). Lichen sclerosus diet: what to eat and avoid. Livestrong.com. https://www.livestrong.com/article/535308-foods-to-avoid-with-lichen-sclerosus/

Website, N. (2024, December 16). Lichen sclerosus. nhs.uk. https://www.nhs.uk/conditions/lichen-sclerosus/

www.ingramcontent.com/pod-product-compliance
Lightning Source LLC
LaVergne TN
LVHW012031060526
838201LV00061B/4555